# AIDS DEMENTIA

## & HIV BRAIN IMPAIRMENT

**Dr. Agnes Kocsis**

St. Mary's Hospital, Paddington

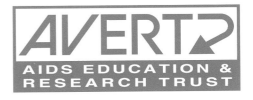

**AVERT**

**AIDS EDUCATION &
RESEARCH TRUST**

# CONTENTS

# INTRODUCTION

This book is primarily for anyone who works in a professional capacity with people with HIV Related Brain Impairment. It is also hoped that partners, family or friends of those with HIV Brain Impairment may find the facts and approaches outlined of value. If you are HIV seropositive yourself and are concerned about brain effects you will hopefully find not only information but some reassurance.

The first section of the book provides an overview of the definition, diagnosis and treatment of HIV Related Brain Impairment. The second section describes assessment and management approaches that can be adopted as part of an approach to good service delivery.

# SECTION 1:

## HOW DOES HIV AFFECT THE BRAIN?

HIV can directly invade the brain and spinal cord (that is the Central Nervous System or CNS). It is probably carried into the brain by monocytes, cells which are produced in the bone marrow and pass into the blood. These cells become macrophages and are present in the brain. HIV directly infects only the white matter of the brain (the glial or 'glue' cells). HIV is able to infect these cells directly just as it is able to infect the CD4 (T-cells) of the immune system. Although it cannot directly invade the neurons, which are the 'thinking' cells of the brain, it appears that the neurons are nevertheless destroyed by indirect means.

There are many hypotheses about the mechanisms for this, but whatever the exact mechanism, it is clear that HIV can cause brain damage which can be progressive and, potentially, irreversible. It is also the case that only damage to the neurons is in principle irreversible, whereas white matter can regenerate. It is also known that the mere presence of HIV in the Central Nervous System (CNS), as shown by finding the virus in the fluid that surrounds the brain and spinal cord (Cerebrospinal Fluid or CSF) is in itself not enough to cause dementia.

Fortunately, the majority of people with HIV do not develop AIDS Dementia, or indeed any level of HIV Brain Impairment. Figures of 10-16% for AIDS Dementia are based on large prevalence studies in the USA. Similar figures emerge from smaller European studies. It is likely that a higher percentage of individuals with HIV have some viral activity in their brain, but this may not necessarily impact on their normal functioning. With the advent of new treatment approaches, it is possible that it will be advantageous to identify those with any level of HIV activity in the brain in order to identify the appropriate treatment. However we are not yet at this stage.

It may also be worth bearing in mind that CNS involvement in HIV is an AIDS defining diagnosis, although HIV Brain Impairment which cannot be categorised as a dementia is perhaps equivocal in this regard.

# THE DEFINITION OF AIDS DEMENTIA & HIV BRAIN IMPAIRMENT

There are a number of terms which are used to refer to the effect of HIV in the CNS. The main ones are as follows:

AIDS Dementia Complex

HIV/AIDS (Related) Dementia

HIV/AIDS Encephalopathy

HIV/AIDS Cognitive Impairment

HIV/AIDS (Related) Brain Impairment

It is useful to be clear about these terms as 'dementia' is a diagnosis which refers to impairment of cognitive functioning (i.e. thinking) severe enough to interfere with social and occupational functioning. The diagnosis includes the idea that it is progressive (i.e. it is a deteriorating condition) and irreversible. The diagnosis of a dementia depends on observations of behaviour. For example, seeing that someone is incapable of looking after themselves and their affairs because of an inability to reason, remember or communicate clearly, and finding no illness or life situation that would explain it. Thus it is impossible to diagnose someone who 'appears normal' as having dementia.

In the case of HIV, the term 'dementia' has been somewhat controversial and can be misleading. Not everyone who has HIV affecting their brain has a 'dementia' and indeed they may never progress to a state as profound as this. However, there is no simple and generally recognised term to refer to difficulties which are not as severe but of the same type. The gradations 'mild', 'moderate' and 'severe' are quite frequently used, but it must be acknowledged that 'mild' dementia can be a contradiction in terms. Nor is it necessarily progressive, nor even irreversible. For all these reasons therefore, the more general term HIV Related Brain Impairment, or even more simply, HIV Brain Impairment, is more appropriate and is used throughout this book. Where the term AIDS Dementia is used, then it is to emphasise the extreme end of the spectrum where there is a definite dementia.

'AIDS Dementia Complex' is a term first used by doctors Navia and Price from the United States, and it is rather less in use currently, at least in the UK. The word 'complex' was added to emphasise that there are three main aspects of the deterioration associated with HIV. That is, not just changes in personality and cognition, but also in motor (physical) functioning. This latter aspect refers to slowing and the tremor and clumsiness which may, but does not always, accompany the other changes.

'Encephalopathy' refers not to observable behaviour but to the brain states underlying dementia and brain impairment. It means literally 'pathology/disease of the brain' and is diagnosed on the basis of brain changes observed by brain scan, brain biopsy or post-mortem brain investigations. In the case of HIV it may be impossible to detect the encephalopathy underlying the changes evidenced by HIV Brain Impairment. There is no 'AIDS Dementia' or 'HIV Brain Impairment' laboratory marker. For example brain scans, particularly Magnetic Resonance Imaging, may well show up changes in the brains of those with AIDS Dementia, but will not always do so, and are therefore not diagnostic.

The only way of diagnosing HIV Brain Impairment is by excluding other diagnoses and assessing the person's behaviour, cognitive and personality changes. If the condition falls short of a true dementia, it will be necessary, at least for diagnostic purposes, to carry out a neuropsychological assessment of the person's reasoning, attention, verbal and spatial abilities, memory capacity, etc. Impairment in these areas is referred to under the umbrella term, 'cognitive impairment'.

# DRUG TREATMENT

Until recently there has been no definite treatment for an individual with HIV Brain Impairment. There is some hope that this may change with the advent of the new treatment approaches to HIV but currently there is no clear evidence for efficacious treatment.

One of the critical issues with drug therapy is the extent to which a given drug can pass the 'blood-brain' barrier. This is just what the name suggests – a barrier which normally protects the CNS from invasion by toxic substances. It is thought that if a drug is to effect levels of HIV in the brain, it will be necessary for the drug to cross the blood-brain barrier. Whether it crosses or not is measured by levels of the drug in the CSF.

There are currently three classes of drugs which are being used or are in trial to treat HIV. The first of these in current clinical use are the nucleoside analogues, and only three appear to penetrate CNS significantly, zidovudine (AZT, Retrovir), lamivudine (3TC, Epivir) and stavudine (d4T, Zerit). Of these only zidovudine has so far been thought to have some useful effect in AIDS Dementia. The levels in the CSF are about 20-30% of the levels in blood. Clinical experience suggests that high dose zidovudine is sometimes useful for achieving a 'window' of improvement in those who may be quite confused. However typically the duration of this improvement does not exceed six to nine months. The mechanism for the improvements has also not been clear. It may be that the drug is capable of clearing viral particles or other toxins which contribute to some of the confusion, but this is only speculative.

The other two nucleoside analogues, lamivudine and stavudine, have also been shown in trials to penetrate into the CSF across the blood-brain barrier, although at the time of writing no clear efficacy in relation to HIV Brain Impairment has been established.

The protease inhibitor group of drugs do not achieve CNS penetration, but in the latest class of drugs, the non-nucleoside analogue reverse transcriptase inhibitors, nevirapine (Viramune) does show CNS penetration.

It seems feasible that the reduction in overall viral load (that is the amounts of HIV in the blood at any one time) achieved by combination therapies which may include protease inhibitors, is likely to have an indirect beneficial effect by protecting the immune system and by limiting the amount of virus in the brain as well as anywhere else in the body.

It is currently not at all clear whether improved anti-HIV treatments will prevent HIV Brain Impairment in the longer term, or whether invasion of the brain will be relatively unaffected by the new approaches. It is obviously a time of change and activity in the treatment field and in this area, as with so many aspects of AIDS, professionals as well as people with HIV have to maintain a balance on the tightrope between caution and optimism.

# OPPORTUNIST BRAIN DISEASE IN HIV

HIV in the CNS is of course different from the many opportunist brain diseases which can invade the brain of someone who is HIV seropositive. As HIV weakens the immune system, the brain, like other organs, becomes vulnerable. Typical examples of such opportunist brain diseases infections are, briefly:

- Cerebral Toxoplasmosis, caused by a parasite commonly carried by perhaps 20% of the population without showing itself. It is acquired from eating raw meat or from contact with cat faeces.

- Cryptococcal Meningitis, an inflammation of the membrane covering of the brain. It is caused by a yeast-type fungus.

- Cytomegalovirus (CMV), caused by a virus common in the general population. It can lead to progressive blindness as well as gastro-intestinal upsets if left untreated.

- Progressive Multifocal Leucoencephalopathy (PML), caused by the JC virus, which spreads throughout the white matter of the brain. Its presentation can be rather similar to AIDS Dementia although weakness on one side of the body and rapid deterioration are more typical of PML.

- Brain Lymphomas. The immune suppression accompanying AIDS can affect the body's ability to stop cells multiplying. Sometimes this results in cancer which may attack the brain resulting in brain tumours.

It is absolutely essential to differentiate HIV Brain Impairment from the opportunist brain diseases. This is primarily because the opportunist brain diseases are in the main treatable, although PML and Lymphomas offer a poor prognosis.

The symptoms of someone with an acute brain infection may be similar to someone with HIV Brain Impairment or AIDS Dementia in that there may be confusion, vagueness, headaches, dizziness, etc. However, for many of the diseases there is a significant difference in that the person is more likely to have other signs of infection such as pyrexia, although in the case of Brain Lymphoma there may be no other overt signs. A differential diagnosis can be made on the basis of a number of investigations, including CSF examination and brain scans which are sensitive to markers of these diseases, even though they do not directly provide information about the presence of HIV in the brain. Thus HIV Brain Impairment is a diagnosis based on exclusion.

# THE PRESENTATION OF HIV BRAIN IMPAIRMENT

In considering the effect of HIV in the CNS it is worth bearing in mind the extent to which not only our thinking or 'cognition', but many aspects of our behaviour, mood and personality are dependent on the state of the brain. The presence of HIV in the brain can therefore directly or indirectly result in extreme changes in mood as well as in confusion, disorientation and disinhibited behaviour.

It is convenient to divide up the effects into those on personality (the person's underlying mood and characteristics), behaviour, and cognition. Also it is worth dividing the types of presentation into two main categories – one of which is characterised by the person becoming 'high' and disinhibited, and the other which is more characterised by lack of motivation and 'vagueness'. The two kinds of presentation may happen in the same person at different times. More usually the 'high' presentation is an earlier manifestation of HIV Brain Impairment and the 'low' amotivational state more characteristic of later stages. However this is only clinical impression and so far there is no evidence biologically for these observations. The classification is thus offered merely for convenience.

Of course no one of the following signs should on its own be taken as a sign of HIV Brain Impairment. In assessment one is looking for significant changes in behaviour (one person's memory problem is another's ordinary absent-mindedness), and a pattern of changes – that is, not placing reliance on just one change.

It cannot be emphasised too strongly that in the matter of assessment and diagnosis, great care must be taken to consider other, or additional, possible reasons for the perceived changes. Neuropsychological assessment should be used to test out the possibility of HIV Related Brain Impairment, and the assessment should also be made in the broader context of the individual's history and cultural context.

In the 'high' presentation some of the following may be observed:

The person may be

- more talkative than usual;

- centred more than usual on immediately reinforcing behaviours such as atypically (and without appropriate funds) spending money on luxury items, ordering expansively from catalogues, etc.;

- more agitated and finding it difficult to concentrate on any one thing, hopping from activity to activity and/or subject to subject;

- more impractical in making plans;

- more careless with personal hygiene, appearance;

- more inappropriate socially (e.g. inappropriate sexual advances, uncharacteristically rude personal remarks, odd style of dress);

- more excessive and exaggerated in making complaints or demands.

In a minority of cases – perhaps one in a hundred people with HIV, the above changes become greatly exaggerated and activity of HIV in the CNS announces itself through a 'psychotic breakdown'. This is probably the result of neurotransmitter abnormalities in the brain caused by the presence of HIV. The episode should be treated as an indicator of possible CNS involvement and once the psychosis has resolved the person will need to be fully assessed.

In the 'low' presentation, the following are typical:

The person may have

- reduced motivation, not accompanied by signs of depression – that is a 'flat' effect without expression of sadness, guilt or fear of the future, etc.;

- a new and marked discrepancy between expressed wish or attitude and action (e.g. "I am quite happy to get out and about" but does not put a foot outside home);

- a reduction in the ability to find the right word, reduced speech output, speaks 'when spoken to';

- slowing of speech, action, etc., not attributable to low mood, fatigue or physical illness;

- reduced concern about personal affairs, future, etc., again in the absence of depressed mood or hopelessness;

- a change in overall levels of arousal and/or biological rhythms (e.g. changed sleeping pattern with sleeplessness at night and sleepiness during the day, decreased appetite not resulting from mood disturbance or physical causes, loss of interest in sex for no physical or emotional reasons);

- increased vagueness, (poorer descriptions, less specific about details of events, etc.) new and marked indecisiveness, perhaps resulting in lack of action;

- poorer memory, particularly problems in remembering past events and in remembering very familiar names;

- reading and writing difficulties in terms of either motor difficulties or formulation of sentences.

## THE NATURE OF HIV RELATED BRAIN IMPAIRMENT (COGNITIVE DIFFICULTIES)

In most cases of HIV Brain Impairment and AIDS Dementia, the essence of 'who the person is' is preserved, and memory problems are usually not as central as with other types of dementia. The primary difficulty is with attention – that is being able to screen out distractions, carrying out tasks which require several stages for completion, and 'dual-tasking' where two competing activities need to be carried out simultaneously (driving and arguing might be an example!).

In addition motor tasks requiring precision (typing, playing an instrument, writing, etc.) become particularly difficult where, rather than the task being automatic, there is a demand to 'think' as well. Typing a difficult letter, writing out accounts, learning a new instrumental piece, might all be examples. Typically also the person will be slowed down, although to varying extents and this might not be noticeable in everyday functioning at all, even if it is apparent on neuropsychological testing.

The difficulty with concentration and 'keeping on track', results in a number of difficulties. The essence of these is the lowered threshold for distractibility. While normally the person would be able to start an activity and then, after answering the phone or going to the toilet return to continue it, it is much more likely that the interruption will drive out the 'sense of purpose'. This is the kind of problem that results in pans burning, appointments being forgotten and letters remaining half-written. It also leaves the individual feeling chaotic and out of control with a – quite realistic – feeling of not being able to 'get things done'. In addition, partners and family are bound to feel the effects of these changes. The more responsibilities held by the individual, the more impact this type of problem will have on the lives of others.

Other ways in which the cognitive difficulties may manifest themselves include the inability to get absorbed in film or television programmes (due to 'losing the thread') and a problem with attending to more than one person talking and hence a dislike of larger groups.

There may be considerable difficulty with concentration, especially with unfamiliar items and following through on actions with several parts (e.g. cooking, letter writing, keeping track of financial affairs).

There may be memory difficulties for behaviours linked to particular dates or times of day (appointments, taking medication, birthdays), and where one is in a particular chain of actions (e.g. "Why am I in this room?"; "What have I been doing for the last while?"). In more severe instances autobiographical memory (for the events of one's life) may also deteriorate.

It is also important to consider the psychological consequences of these difficulties. Unless compensated for, either by strategies or by the intervention of say a partner, the person is almost certain to feel less effective, to be doing less that is satisfying and to be feeling out of control. So it is important for professionals to bear in mind that the person may wish to only interact with familiar people, to only go to familiar places, and they may wish to avoid discussion of their failings and minimise their difficulties so as to avoid humiliation.

In addition the person is likely to prefer to deal with a limited number of decisions and not to be pressured to make quick decisions – for example, about care packages. While accommodating these points is easier said than done, a good service for this group cannot ignore the nature of the specific difficulties experienced.

In addition, if the patient has relatives, a partner or other immediate carers, it will be important to explore how the changes have impacted on their lives together. Sometimes for instance carers take on more and more of the practical organising of life simply because they 'have to' – without really realising the cause of the changes.

# PROVIDING HELP FOR SOMEONE WITH COGNITIVE DIFFICULTIES

There is some general guidance which can be adapted for use with someone with AIDS Dementia who is confused and perhaps whose behaviour is not appropriate to a given situation. The general guidance can also be more specifically adapted in relation to treatment and drug compliance issues.

## GENERAL GUIDELINES

- The person's distractibility can be an advantage – "Come and look at the interesting…"; "Would it be a good idea to have some coffee now?" etc.

- Offer simple, manageable, closed decisions (this or that).

- Make structures and routines clear without being dogmatic. "The doctor comes round at 11 every morning – on Mondays and Thursdays she will see you. You can smoke on the balcony, not in your room".

- Keep repeating timetables and forthcoming events in the flow of conversation so that it does not sound automated but serves as a reassuring reminder of what to expect.

- Never create 'rush'. "The car will be here in ten minutes, do hurry" will only lead to a panic. "Let me find your bag and keys while you get your coat" may be better.

- Sometimes what the person says may be more a request for attention or a way of expressing unhappiness. Unfortunately these efforts are sometimes labelled 'manipulative'. While it is not appropriate for staff or indeed for immediate carers to be manipulated into say, neglecting other duties, some thought about other, structured ways of meeting the person's needs can be more valuable than a 'label'.

- A person with AIDS Dementia generally has unimpaired social skills and is responsive to the nuances of social interaction. Thus genuine respect, courtesy and humour where appropriate will oil interactions as they generally do. If these fail, because the person is angry or frustrated and irritable, it may be better to withdraw so that this can pass away. A person with HIV Brain Impairment who is frequently 'flying off the handle' should be treated as being overly stressed by current circumstances. Maybe there are too many demands or too little predictability.

## TREATMENT AND DRUG COMPLIANCE ISSUES

### In the Outpatient Clinic

With the advent of new treatment approaches to HIV which are associated with complex pill-taking regimes, there will at times be concern about the ability of people with HIV Brain Impairment to decide about and adhere to treatment. Whereas the person with cognitive difficulties can make decisions appropriately in most cases, not too much choice should be offered.

For everyone involved with HIV the current barrage of sometimes conflicting information is hard to process and generates feelings of uncertainty. For someone with HIV Brain Impairment the clinician will need to process the possible options to the minimum before presenting them to the person concerned. It is also quite typical of the type of cognitive impairment associated with HIV, for the individual to get distracted from the main question at hand by a number of peripheral issues – say, the size of the pills or whether there will be drinking water available at the day centre. This may be to the exclusion of the general issue of whether the treatment is likely to be efficacious.

Once a decision to take treatment has been made, it has to be reviewed on a frequent basis, probably weekly until the regime is established. There are a number of electronic devices which can help to prompt a person to take medication. Apart from electronic organisers there exist various beeper systems, some of which can take messages from a central source.

So a poor memory is not a reason for not taking combination therapy, although provision of a beeper is also not a sufficient reason for assuming that the problems of compliance have been solved. Strategies for 'following through' on taking the medication once there has been a reminder will need to be established. It would probably be appropriate for the patient to be able to have guidance on these issues from someone who can be fairly freely available, especially in the early days of taking the therapy, and who understands how to implement remedial strategies in this area.

### On the Ward

For patients with HIV Brain Impairment treatment decisions should, as in the outpatient clinic, be treated with particular care as any sort of systemic illness may exacerbate existing cognitive difficulties. Pneumocystis Carinii Pneumonia (PCP) for example may deplete the brain of oxygen resulting in confusion. Liver or kidney infections can result in a toxic confusional state and steroidal treatments for example can lead to an apparent psychosis. In fact in clinical experience it appears that those with an existing brain vulnerability may first evidence impairment to others around them at the time of such episodes. In any case it is wise to ensure that all important treatment issues are discussed with the same person and only that person; that information (facts, times of investigations etc.) is recorded in a bedside notebook and that immediate carers are fully informed so that they feel in a good position to back up information from the doctors and nurses.

In the case of someone with AIDS Dementia or with a psychotic episode resulting from HIV activity in the brain, the ward staff may find it helpful to use some of the general guidelines mentioned above. Although it is very helpful to have the skills of mental health trained nurses, this group of patients have an organic condition causing their difficulties and it is important to bear this in mind.

# SECTION 2:

## INITIATING ASSESSMENTS

For a service to be offered to those with HIV Brain Impairment, a necessary first step is diagnosis on the basis of assessment. While the point is a simple one, this first step may not be so simple and there are a number of different matters to consider.

While professionals working in GUM, 'Special Clinics' and HIV specialist centres are generally comfortable in talking about death and the details of sexual behaviour – both subjects with their own 'taboos' – the subject of dementia may be less familiar. Given this fear of the unknown, together with a very natural belief that dementia is an appalling catastrophe involving total humiliation and loss of control, it is hardly surprising that a major factor in assessment delay is the reluctance of everyone concerned to raise the possibility of brain impairment with the person concerned.

Where problems are referred to by the patient, or by someone in the patient's immediate network, professionals have at least implicit 'permission' to carry out a complete assessment. However one cannot rely on this happening. If a patient does not self refer, but has personality, behaviour or cognition changes observed by others it may be up to a responsible professional to initiate the assessment process.

Initiating the process is easier if the professional concerned is aware of the necessary procedures and if the potential value of assessment is clear. There is no point in diagnosing brain impairment if there can be no follow-up of any sort – no support, no advice, no access to practical help or potential treatment. However since this is unlikely to be the case, at least in most Western centres specialising in HIV treatment, it is essential to recognise that ignoring HIV Brain Impairment is poor, if not negligent, practice.

There are some considerable advantages to a timely assessment which include:

- A great deal of support can be offered to improve the quality of the person's life by offering practical help geared to the cognitive and psychological needs raised by brain impairment. It is not unusual for someone who receives such support to have a much improved sense of well-being and to feel much better 'cognitively' by having life simplified.

- The person concerned can take much more control and can communicate to everyone concerned their preferences for treatment, housing, support, etc. as well as being able to arrange personal affairs such as a will.

- The person concerned should hopefully have an opportunity to talk through psychological issues and be able to build up a relationship with one or more people who will later be 'key' in arranging care and other services.

- The person's partner, relatives and friends can be offered a framework for understanding the reason for changes of mood, distractibility or impetuousness. This can avoid some of the sheer distress and emotional confusion which the change in someone they love can arouse and gives them access to information and support.

- If in addition the person concerned has dependants, then it is incumbent on the professionals involved to proceed with assessment lest, for example, children come to be at risk.

## A SHARED FRAMEWORK

Differing viewpoints are also a frequent barrier to the instigation of assessment. It can be onerous for someone to initiate assessment if other staff members or other parts of the local HIV service do not share a framework of understanding about HIV Brain Impairment. Depending on factors such as experience, knowledge of mental health issues, familiarity with the patient and feelings about brain impairment, different professionals may have quite diverse perceptions of the problems presented by a patient.

For example, in someone with a history of alcohol or drug use, or of psychiatric difficulties or indeed if someone is under acute stress, personality changes may be attributed entirely to these other factors. However, one has to bear in mind that a diagnosis of depression or a history of drug use is no barrier to HIV Related Brain Impairment. It is certainly possible to have one as well as the other. In the case of those with a history of previous brain insult there is evidence to suggest that they may be more, rather than less vulnerable to HIV Brain Impairment. Assessment in these cases may be especially complex but will nevertheless need to be addressed.

To achieve this 'shared framework' it is helpful if within HIV services professionals can work together to establish referral routes and assessment procedures as well as adopting service guidelines. Such work can prevent cases 'slipping through the net' in such a way that diagnosis is only made late on when the person is suffering from severe AIDS Dementia, and probably causing difficulties for care managers and hospital staff as well as for their informal carers.

In settings where HIV infected parents and children are seen separately by adult and paediatric HIV services, much thought should be given to the communication between the two. It is essential that all professionals are fully informed if there is HIV Brain Impairment in a parent, since it is not unusual for a psychotic episode, disinhibited or careless behaviour to leave a child at risk. This is a situation where the parent cannot be held responsible and support for a family in good time should ensure that no drastic procedures, such as taking a child into care, are invoked.

Of course in the case of some families who have come to the UK either as refugees or as immigrants, the perception of statutory services may be such that they are fearful of discussing their concerns. Much sensitivity, persistence and the use of local networks may be required to establish trust – however a service can work to gain a reputation for reliability and again, this is much more likely to be the case when crises are avoided and HIV Related Brain Impairment is diagnosed earlier rather than later.

## ASSESSMENT APPROACHES

There are a number of different stages in the assessment process, and these are basically as follows:

1 Exclusion of opportunist infection or other systemic infection;

2 Information on other factors potentially affecting cognition, e.g. drug and alcohol misuse, past head injury, ischaemic conditions;

3 Information from carers on any changes observed in personality, behaviour and cognition;

4 Assessment of mood, personality and any psychiatric history;

5 Neuropsychological testing;

6 Activities of Daily Living Interview;

7 Activities of Daily Living Observation.

Generally it is not until problems are apparent that assessment approaches are implemented. However there are many advantages in having a baseline assessment as part of the initial clinical workup. This is particularly so for anyone who might present confounding factors in an assessment procedure. For example those who:

• do not speak English as their mother tongue;

• come from a culture which may be misunderstood by the local medical services;

• have a history of brain insult (due to trauma, alcohol or drugs misuse, etc.);

• may have other factors affecting brain functioning (e.g. epilepsy, learning disability, age related decline);

• have a history of major psychiatric disorder.

In these cases, a baseline assessment of mood state and cognition through neuropsychological assessment allows any change to be documented in a straightforward fashion. Having baseline assessment as routine can also help if a potential referrer finds difficulty in raising the possibility of brain impairment with an individual.

## ACTIVITIES OF DAILY LIVING – METHODS OF GAINING INFORMATION

Respect for individuals with brain impairment is not the same thing as assuming that their verbal, subjective reports of what they can and cannot do is accurate or necessarily gives the full picture without prompting. In other words it is not enough to ask "Can you cook for yourself?". "Of course I can!" could be true in the sense that with prompting the person will make toast and coffee. It does not give any idea about whether the person is able to plan a meal, shop for it, feel motivated to get round to preparing it and then be able to carry that through without getting distracted.

Considering whether a parent with brain impairment is likely to be able to cook appropriately for children will be even more complex. On the other hand it is possible to improve the quality of information the patient can provide by keeping the questions specific and keeping them in context. Thus it may be easier to find out details by starting with a very specific question such as 'What did you eat yesterday?' or 'What do your kids like best to eat?' There are provisos of course – memory and verbal difficulties will influence people's ability to answer these questions. Other sources of information such as immediate carers will be necessary to complete the picture.

## GIVING THE DIAGNOSIS

It is important that when diagnosing someone as having HIV Brain Impairment the following information is conveyed, in order that the diagnosis is not seen as necessarily being catastrophic:

- A diagnosis of HIV Brain Impairment indicates HIV activity in the brain. It is not necessarily a diagnosis of 'dementia';

- The person's state will not necessarily deteriorate, especially in the early stages. Given the changing picture with treatments, optimism is not inappropriate;

- The person's basic intelligence is not affected, at least only in a few cases and then in very extreme states. The difficulties experienced with attention, concentration, motivation, etc. (see below) can often be compensated for. Thus the person need not think of themselves as becoming 'stupid'.

# THE CONSEQUENCES OF A DIAGNOSIS OF HIV BRAIN IMPAIRMENT

Once a diagnosis has been made it is essential that feedback and the option of follow-up advice and support is given to the patient, and if possible and appropriate to the immediate carer(s). This should include an exploration of any currently perceived difficulties on either side.

The patient and carers should be given separate time to discuss their concerns and feelings. It is wise to acknowledge that our understanding of the way in which HIV Brain Impairment progresses and might be treated is still poor. Over time, rather than in the first feedback session, it will be possible to explore some useful planning strategies. For example for anyone with possible brain impairment it will be necessary to consider:

- Appointing Power of Attorney. This allows the person to choose someone who would act in financial matters should this become necessary. Once the forms for indicating who would be chosen to act are completed, there is no reason to do any more unless the person does indeed become quite incapable of handling financial issues. The Power of Attorney can then be activated by sending in the form. Details can be obtained from the Public Trust Office.

- Arranging a Will. This of course is not particular to someone with brain impairment. However sometimes people feel that they would rather wait until the last possible moment before making a will. A diagnosis of brain impairment may prompt them to act earlier.

- Considering other preferences that others should be aware of. Treatment choices as well as care choices might be relevant here, including who might need to be excluded from visiting or taking a major role in care if the person is no longer able to communicate wishes.

Tentatively it might also be worth granting permission for certain constraining actions at a later date. Those who drink or use drugs heavily are at risk of an exacerbation of addictive behaviour with AIDS Dementia. This often poses a great ethical problem for carers, professional and personal. If a person felt able, for example, to state that it would be acceptable to withhold such substances if consumption was a danger, it might facilitate management later.

The way of accessing support and a description of some of the issues which may emerge can be useful. Immediate carers particularly value telephone access to discuss problematic issues as they arise. 'Safety versus independence' and 'letting be versus stimulation' can be salient issues for instance. Carers may need 'permission' to discuss these concerns and highlighting areas that others have needed to talk about can be a good way of doing this. Of course the availability of services will also need to be explored, although it is perhaps preferable to wait a little before offering too many options.

# THE PHILOSOPHY OF SERVICE PROVISION

It is important to consider the purpose of services for people with HIV Brain Impairment and the 'spirit' in which they are offered.

## THE AIMS OF INTERVENTIONS

It is probably true to say that ten years ago, people with HIV Brain Impairment tended to be identified only at the stage when they had developed AIDS Dementia, and then perhaps only at the stage where they had a short while to live, perhaps a few weeks or months. The aim at that time was primarily to make them comfortable and support their carers.

However as awareness of HIV Brain Impairment has increased and assessment methods have improved, and as HIV treatments have prolonged people's lives, the expectations about the aims of input with this client group have also changed. Essentially it is now possible to think in terms of rehabilitation – that is of offering people with HIV Brain Impairment the possibility of improvement, rather than deterioration, through the structured teaching of strategies and other aids. However, the goals that can be set with any one individual will of course differ according to the level of impairment observed.

A central idea in the rehabilitation of people with HIV Brain Impairment is that of allowing life to continue in as normal a way as possible. Rather than introducing new activities and lifestyles, maximising their ability to continue previously preferred activities appears to be more acceptable.

One concept that can be helpful in this regard is that of JEST (Just Enough Support for the Task). JEST prioritises the goal of considering what would be required to allow the person to continue to carry out specific tasks or activities. Sometimes it is assumed by the person themselves as well as their own carers, that if it is not possible to do something the way it was previously done, then it is not possible at all.

An example of JEST is that of a person who lacks 'get up and go' and can therefore no longer be 'bothered' to go swimming. Providing a taxi and a suitable companion might be enough to make the difference.

However JEST need not always be in the form of a companion. It may be in the form of helping the person to establish a habit or define a structure which, for example, allows activities to be carried out in spite of the distractibility which has been highlighted as a central feature of HIV related cognitive impairment.

There are a number of different strategies which can help and one example is that of 'chunking' activities.

What this means is that for someone with normal attention it is often possible to carry out more than one activity quasi-simultaneously. The tasks will be 'chunked' as separate, even though they may interweave with one another. For example a parent may be preparing breakfast, helping to get the children dressed and getting things ready for work at the 'same' time by doing elements of each in turn (cleaning the shoes while the toast browns, say).

With HIV Brain Impairment this is not an efficient strategy and the person must learn to 'chunk' activities leading towards a particular goal, such that they form a totally predictable set of activities with one leading inevitably to the next with no irrelevant activity allowed to intrude. This idea in itself will, at least in the early stages, be easy for the person to grasp and be appreciated as quite applicable.

It is of course important to separate out this aspect of tasks from the memory aspect. That is, remembering to begin an activity is one thing, which can be prompted in a number of different ways. Remembering to follow through on the activity however, is another. This can best be established initially by making a checklist, and asking the patient to identify a given order of carrying out the checks so that a routine is established.

## PSYCHIATRIC LIAISON

As already explained, HIV activity in the brain sometimes manifests as a psychotic episode. In the case of someone who has had no psychiatric history previous to HIV, and in whom the psychotic episode does not appear to have any link to life events, it is possible to diagnose HIV CNS involvement as causative of the episode. In this sense, the 'psychiatric' episode is essentially as much a part of the organic features of HIV as, say, involvement of the lymph nodes. Due however to Western medicine's emphasis on the 'body-mind' disjunction, the personality alterations caused by HIV in the brain may have to be treated by a different set of services, i.e. the psychiatric services as opposed to HIV services.

The practical difficulty arising out of this anomaly is that while HIV services at the time of writing are still not catchment bound, psychiatric services are. Thus a patient may be receiving HIV services out of catchment area, but be obliged to receive psychiatric input locally. This makes liaison very difficult, with particular dilemmas where the patient is also 'ill in body' in more obvious ways.

The most effective answer is to have good HIV psychiatric liaison, with attached beds, for anyone who needs to be treated voluntarily or involuntarily sectioned under the Mental Health Act. If this is not possible, then having nurses with mental health interest, if not experience, on medical wards dealing with people with HIV can be advantageous. It appears to be the case that often there are particular medical nurses who develop an interest and skill in dealing with HIV Brain Impaired patients, and can with the support of psychology and psychiatry, help to support someone with an HIV related psychiatric episode on the medical ward. Resources are necessary to allow the patient to be 'specialled' for at least some days on the ward, given that an agitated, wandering and disinhibited individual can not only wander off the ward but may at times disturb others.

With careful observation of the milder symptoms of personality change, it may be possible to predict an imminent hypomanic or paranoid psychotic episode and avoid or minimise it through prescription of a low dose of a major tranquilliser such as 'Serenace' (haloperidol). Obviously, people who know the patient well are much more likely to be sensitive to the degree of such personality changes and may need to keep careful notes of the changes observed to be able to report these back to the patient's clinician or psychiatrist. Avoidance of the type of breakdown which results in voluntary, or more frequently involuntary, admission for psychiatric treatment is obviously preferable, for the immediate carers as much as for the patient concerned.

Carers may totally lose their trust in HIV services if their partner, child or friend is forced into a unit which is for 'mad' people. They may have their own experiences of psychiatric services which prejudices them against all such interventions and the patient's own perception of what is happening can be coloured by such attitudes which can feed into paranoid ideation.

For this reason, if for no other, it is very helpful to be able to explain to patients and to carers before symptoms get extreme, what the possible scenarios might be if things progress.

# CARE PACKAGES & COMMUNITY PROVISION

## CARE PACKAGES

The planning of care packages for people with HIV Brain Impairment can be challenging, even where there are resources available. There are a number of reasons for this including:

- Services may be limited and lack flexibility of response;

- Patients may refuse services;

- HIV Brain Impaired patients may be particularly intolerant of unpredictability, changing staff or the occasional 'faux pas';

- Resources for providing the infrastructure to allow services to be used well (e.g. transport) may not be available.

It can be a challenge for carers to establish and maintain the 'right note' in their relationship with patients. The essence of this is to find the point which maximises professional competence on the one hand and human 'care' (in the real sense of the word) on the other. Such a relationship opens channels of communication with the patient which is likely to mean that the services offered are best matched to the patient's needs and wishes.

In the case of people with brain impairment this may be hard, perhaps because frequently carers are required to control the patient's behaviour in various ways. Carers may also feel upset by a patient and, occasionally, afraid. In order to get round these difficulties carers may choose to adopt a stance which emphasises the professional-patient distance. There are many ways of achieving this – extreme efficiency, 'exaggerated' patience and the brisk 'no-nonsense' approach being among them. All of these have a place within the repertoire of professional behaviour and are essential with 'borderline' patients or those who are unable to respond to 'give and take' in their interactions with services. However these approaches may be counterproductive with other patients who need to establish trust in professional carers if they are to make best use of what is on offer.

Carers need to feel confident that the approach they use matches the needs of the situation and the patient at the time. Training and backup are required to ensure that carers are definite about their role and have the necessary professional skills.

Paradoxically, more experienced and confident carers are better able to establish personal and warm relationships with patients without compromising their professional role. Professional-personal boundaries are much less likely to 'blur' if the carer is certain about the tasks required by the professional role.

## GOOD FOUNDATIONS

Most care packages stand or fall according to the solidity of their foundations. These foundations are the type of relationship between the person concerned and the carers – individually and as a group. For these to be well prepared it is generally an advantage to have at least some of the following:

- gradual introduction to whatever services are to be used;

- use of 'bridges' provided by people who are already known and trusted by the person concerned;

- concentration in the first hours or days on forming a relationship with the person concerned. For planning and resource purposes, this means that more time may need to be allocated in the early days, so that there is less sense of hurry, e.g. to get a meal prepared in a home setting or to move on with the tasks of the group in a day care environment.

## MAINTAINING AUTONOMY AND DECISION-MAKING

One of the frustrations for someone with brain impairment is likely to be a sense of decreased autonomy. To counteract this, and to ensure a care package does not break down due to 'spilling over' of this frustration, it is vital to avoid 'taking over' although how to avoid this can often be a puzzle – "If he cannot choose where to go, or always chooses something unrealistic, what shall we do?"

One possibility is to have in mind the general rule 'How can a decision be offered which is manageable?' Thus, for example, it may be possible to point to just two possible choices, say "Would you prefer to listen to this CD or that one?" (Instead of "What would you like to do now?") or "Do you want to ring so-and-so now or after lunch?" (Instead of "What are you going to do about contacting your social worker?").

Naturally all carers, whether professionals or not, worry about taking away someone's freedom to make decisions. The right to choose treatment and services is the essence of the notion of 'empowerment'. In dealing with individuals with brain impairment it is important that the spirit, rather than the letter, of this notion is adhered to. For example, it is not 'empowerment' to ask someone with brain impairment "Do you want someone to come in to your house three times a week?" and accept "No" for an answer without question.

Empowering people with HIV Brain Impairment to make decisions means ensuring that the choices they are offered and the way in which they are offered these choices is suited to their cognitive capacity. Thus it is likely to be necessary to pursue the question in much more detail. Once you get down to specifics, the reasons for the reluctance are bound to become clearer and a solution may become obvious.

Of course offers of service are often refused for 'emotional' reasons and as important as acknowledging the cognitive difficulties is to ensure that choices are offered in a way which acknowledges the psychological state of the person with HIV Brain Impairment. Thus if someone is confused, that individual will crave familiarity and is likely to find unfamiliar people and situations threatening. Similarly an individual who is struggling with a sense of incompetence and loss of control will be threatened by the professional competency and 'briskness' of some service organisations.

## HOME CARE ISSUES

Obviously home care staff need to be very sensitive to the possible sense of intrusion associated with being in someone else's 'space' – however much the person appears to need assistance. Unfortunately, in most cases little specific training is offered to staff attending people with HIV Brain Impairment, and thus misunderstandings arise which result in tearful and vituperous collapse of care packages.

It is obviously ideal if staff can be trained to assess tasks and plan JEST strategies. In particular they can be helpful in supporting the person to establish constructive habits and routines. If this is done thoughtfully and without undue haste, using immediate carers to bridge the 'unfamiliarity gap' it should be possible to avoid many of the situations where the carer is left standing at the door refused entry.

In addition home care staff should have training to allow them to observe possible deterioration or previously unnoticed areas of difficulty and they should know how to feed these back appropriately. Again the daily contact with a skilled home care person can prevent collapse of the care package.

## DAY OCCUPATION – PURPOSE AND ORGANISATION

In thinking of day occupation the overall purposes of intervention will again be important. For example, keeping in mind the goal of rehabilitation, day occupation may be presented not just as 'filling the time' but as learning to move towards greater independence through compensating for some of the difficulties in daily living. It may also be possible to offer a structure for someone's day which they can learn to adopt as a way of life, and which will allow more control and independence. In the light of this it may often be useful to involve a partner or other immediate carer in the activities if this is possible.

One of the major problems for someone with HIV Brain Impairment is simply boredom as concentration difficulties mean that previously enjoyed activities such as reading, writing, watching films, cooking elaborate meals and, of course, most paid occupations become less satisfying.

With the deprivation of these enjoyments as well as of the social benefits these activities may offer, life can seem quite boring and purposeless. As pointed out above, HIV Brain Impairment is perfectly compatible with a high level of intelligence. Nor do skills in themselves necessarily deteriorate. Occupations offered therefore do not have to be 'simple' – rather they need to be offered in such a way as to maximise the likelihood of fairly quick satisfaction and a sense of working towards a purpose and of being involved with others.

## MULTIPLE-PROBLEM PATIENTS

A great deal of what has been written above refers to those with mild to moderate HIV Brain Impairment who are otherwise not particularly vulnerable. However it must be acknowledged that increasingly a high proportion of the work of services dealing with the HIV Brain Impaired is focused on multiple-problem patients who pose tremendous difficulties for management. Such patients may have a history of drug and/or alcohol abuse, extensive psychiatric history, etc. It is likely that if such individuals are to achieve real change they need, at least initially, very contained structures which may be achievable only in residential settings. There are as yet unfortunately very few such facilities catering for this challenging group and this is a clear gap in service provision.

# RESOURCES & USEFUL CONTACTS

## FURTHER READING

Price R W and Perry S W (ed.) *HIV, AIDS and the Brain*. Raven Press, 1994.

## ORGANISATIONS

Both the organisations listed below can provide specialised residential care for people with HIV Brain Impairment:

**London Lighthouse**
111–117 Lancaster Road
London W11 1QT
Tel: 0171 792 1200

**Mildmay Mission Hospital**
Hackney Road
London E2 7NA
Tel: 0171 613 6300

## INTERNET SITES

Below are two internet sites that contain recent and relevant information around HIV Brain Impairment. It is worth remembering that such information can date quickly, so visit AVERT's web site at http://www.avert.org/ for links to the most up-to-date sites:

**Cliniweb**
http://www.ohsu.edu/cliniweb/C10/C10.228.140.380.html

**Alzheimer Europe**
http://www.alzheimer-europe.org/aids.html

AVERT and the author would welcome feedback on this book, especially suggestions on successful service delivery packages and management techniques.